In the Space Between Moments

Finding Joy and Meaning in Medicine

Pranay Sinha

To Anne—my boss, my emotional barometer, my wife.

Table of Contents

Introduction   9

1. The Best Christmas Gift I Ever Gave   16

2. The Last Word   28

3. Urine Trouble   37

4. Nails and Screw-ups   47

5. A Burden I Was Happy to Bear   56

6. Yogesh   68

7. An Intern Writes to His Future Self   75

A Final Word   83

Attributions   86

Acknowledgments   87

Cover Design   89

About the Author   90

Note

These accounts are based on my experiences during residency training. I have changed the names and identifying details of the characters in this book to preserve patient confidentiality. In some cases, I have used composite characters or compressed story lines to better convey the narrative and my conclusions.

Introduction

My intern gazed blankly at her notes from the day.

"You OK?" I asked.

Her face was quivering with restrained tears as she turned to me. "I don't think I helped anyone today." This was not the first time, nor would it be the last time, that I had heard those words from a resident physician.

Taking the notes from my intern's hands, I sat down next to her.

"Look," I said, "you gave this young woman the right antibiotics for her kidney infection, and she feels better now."

I started flipping through the notes of all her patients one by one.

"You sent this man back home to his wife and kids who missed him. You reassured this boy's parents that he's going to be fine. You spared this terminally ill lady confusion and unnecessary suffering by helping her understand that her time is coming."

I looked up at her from the notes and said, "Today, you played an important role in all their lives."

The tears refused to be choked back any further, but they were accompanied by a little smile. "Yeah, I guess I did."

****

Unless you live under a rock, you've probably heard that health-care workers worldwide are experiencing a dark phenomenon called burnout. If physician burnout was a stock, you should have invested in the eighties.

A PubMed search of medical literature reveals that there were only seven references to "physician burnout" in 1986. In 2017, there were 316. These numbers don't include the hundreds of articles that reference burnout in non-academic publications, blogs, and the mainstream media.

Here's the thing: I am burned out by all this talk about burnout.

Burnout is a real problem and it must be addressed. I am happy that the growing conversation about it has spurred wellness initiatives across the country. However, well-intentioned conversations on burnout can also enshroud us in billows of despair and cloud our view of our professions and our lives.

After completing medical school in Virginia, I moved up north to begin my residency training at Yale-New Haven Hospital. Although I started with the energy of a lively puppy driven to hypomania by a double shot of espresso, the myriad intellectual, physical, and spiritual challenges of working in the land of the sick and dying got to me.

Even though I laughed loudly in workrooms and wore even louder bow ties, I felt a constant malaise, as if I had the flu without a cough or a fever. I started coming home to brimming glasses of red wine and stacks of articles on burnout from venues ranging from the Kevin MD blog to the *New York Times*. Within three months of my intern year, I wrote my own residency confidential for the *Times* about physician suicide.

Suddenly, I transformed into the "suicide guy." I became a faux pundit, answering questions about life, the universe, and everything. Residents and interns started reaching out to me. Some offered words of comfort. Some vented. Some thought I was a pansy. Many of the people who reached out to me sought the same holy grail: joy. Was the practice of medicine antithetical to joy? Were joy and medicine like Venn diagrams forbidden from intersecting by the laws of man and nature?

Soon I stopped contributing to the conversation on burnout and physician wellness because I felt I didn't have anything original to say. But I privately continued to seek the grail. It was only as a third-year resident, after I had to talk my intern through all she had accomplished during her day, that I realized that something had blinded us to the joy in medicine.

Being in my third decade, I still have physical photo albums. Transparent plastic pockets guard my childhood memories with their lives. I love flipping through the pages, lingering in the afterglow of moments of laughter from decades ago. In my favorite photo, I am three years old, buck naked, and have slathered what seems like an entire can of shaving cream on my face to imitate my father. Dad is suitably amused and gazes on me indulgently.

I pick up the album on slow days when I have time or on days when I need time to slow down. A few seconds lingering over the photos gives me the wherewithal to deal with the routine furor of the hospital.

It strikes me that we don't need photo albums, be they physical or digital. For there is joy in the spaces between the moments that play out in the hospital every single day.

Every surgeon has felt a tiny shiver of delight after nailing a challenging procedure for the first time.

Every nurse has felt uplifted after seeing colleagues do something altruistic for their patients.

Every physician has felt a small jolt of bliss after hearing a sincere "Thank you, doctor."

If only we could train our eyes to linger momentarily over the joy that lies between moments like these. This is joy that could be ours.

Joy that should be ours! Buttressed by a stash of joyful memories, we can better endure the inevitable difficulties of residency. To borrow from Brene Brown: "Joy, collected over time, breeds resilience."

Of course, simply appreciating these moments of joy will not eliminate suffering. There is no denying that our work sometimes depletes us. A positive attitude won't neutralize all unpleasant experiences. There will still be unstoppable deaths, long days, and prickly colleagues. But perhaps an inclination toward finding joy in the midst of difficult moments might make the misery seem less monolithic.

Finding nuggets of happiness in the daily grind of medicine need not be complicated. Everyone has a way. Some practice appreciative inquiry by being curious about the people around them and being prompt with their praise: "That's a cool tattoo. Tell me about it!" or "Did you see how artfully Dr. Wu explained the plan to the patient?" Others may opt for mindfulness, journaling, or poetry. Really, the method is less important than the desire—nay determination—to find joy. And oftentimes we need someone or something to point us in the right direction. And that is why I have written this book.

I hope that these stories will remind all those who devote their lives to caring for others to keep finding joy in the space between moments.

The Best Christmas Gift I Ever Gave

Although it was Christmas eve, cheer was in short supply under the fluorescent lights of the intensive care unit (ICU). It was my last twenty-four-hour call for the month. December had been rough. The flu had wreaked havoc among the elderly and weak. And then there was the steady stream of patients from the oncology floors. An orchestra of unceasing alarms constantly reminded me that these patients were teetering on the precipice of mortality. Some got better. Many didn't.

After rounds, the admitting resident told me I was needed in the Emergency Room (ER). He smiled wryly. "They say she's dead to the world."

"Find her a graveyard," I muttered, as I slunk down to the ER. I immediately felt guilty.

The last month in the ICU had eroded my compassion and curiosity. Unlike other residents, I found no joy in the extremes of human physiology on display in the ICU, just irritation and despair. I wasn't bad at critical care, but neither was I great. Day after day patients seemingly got better or worse regardless of what we, residents, did. The attending physicians called most of the shots anyway.

I found her lying alone in the resuscitation bay. The tubes in her mouth were urging her to go on breathing. The pile of medical debris around her bed testified to the frantic effort to save her.

"*Carol!*" I yelled in her ear over the din of the ventilator, "my name is Dr. Sinha. Don't panic! We'll get you feeling better."

No response. I went through a standard list of barbaric actions that we euphemistically call "noxious stimuli." I pinched her, rubbed her sternum with painful pressure, and pushed hard on her fingernails with my pen. Any one of these "stimuli" can have a Lazarus effect on most lightly sedated people, but she didn't turn a hair.

Mercifully, I didn't see any evidence of gross brain damage. On her left hand, I saw a rather weighty antique gold ring in need of cleaning. In the ICU, fingers often swell up with IV fluids. I took off her ring to safeguard the blood supply to her finger.

The ED resident moseyed over as I was easing the ring off her finger. He sported a leather holster on the waist of his scrubs that held a stethoscope. I wondered if he called himself "Dr. Quick Draw."

"Big stroke," he surmised, tapping his index finger on his right temple. "Shame," he added hastily, perhaps worried about seeming flippant.

"Hmm…certainly possible. Let's keep a broad differential for now," I suggested. "Is the family around?"

Following Dr. Quick Draw's directions, I found Carol's wife, Ann, and mother, Claire, in a small, windowless waiting room. Ann told me the story as Claire nodded.

Carol and Ann had spent the previous evening cooking up a storm for their upcoming Christmas party. Their already cramped kitchen felt even cozier as it filled with laughter and the competing aromas of hot chocolate and apple pie. They ended their night by swapping childhood memories by their fireplace, clinking whiskey glasses and laughing some more.

The next morning, Ann awoke to find Carol still sleeping next to her. A self-confessed "type A personality," Carol had always gotten up, dressed, and cleaned up her email inbox before Ann stumbled out of bed. Today was different.

Ann spent the first minute teasing her but became worried when there was no retort. She started shaking and pinching Carol, first tentatively then frantically. Hearing Ann's screams, Claire called 911.

In the ED, Carol was not breathing well and was intubated. Ann kept asking the physicians about what was going on.

One of the early possibilities that had been suggested was a massive stroke with a poor prognosis. Ann felt her stomach lurch. Carol had been laughing next to the fireplace not twelve hours ago. How could this be? Ann needed to sit down.

There is no new drug, no new gadget that can give a physician the words to comfort a grieving spouse or a bereaved mother. I pressed the ring into Ann's hand and hugged her.

Carol's head CT did not show a stroke. We were in the dark about her sudden unconsciousness. Ann remembered that in addition to her regular medicines, Carol kept a bunch of expired drugs in her bathroom cabinet. Ann drove home to get them while we ordered a tox screen.

By the time she returned, Carol's urine had tested positive for benzodiazepines. The mostly empty bottles Ann brought back confirmed that Carol had been using old prescriptions for Valium.

The story now seemed clearer: the whiskey and Valium combination had knocked Carol unconscious and depressed her breathing to a dangerous degree.

"Do you have an antidote?"

I nodded: "Yes, but it's better to let the drug wear off."

"How long will it take?"

"Difficult to say. Why don't you go home and get some rest? I'll call you if things change."

Reluctantly, Ann got up and stretched. She gazed out at the inky New Haven sky. Then she kissed Carol's forehead, picked up her coat, and began walking out. She stopped and turned to me. "Do you have someone you love?"

I am careful about sharing my personal life with patients, but I could see no harm here.

"Yes, I have a girlfriend. She's pretty special."

"Make sure you kiss her passionately every night. You never know what tomorrow will bring."

During a rushed dinner of Graham crackers and peanut butter, I texted my girlfriend: "FYI—I love you."

"You're a weirdo," she responded.

I didn't have another spare moment after that. The MICU's pace that night was frenetic. I ran from room to room managing ventilator settings, titrating norepinephrine drips, and adjusting sedatives. Around 5:00 a.m., I was summoned to Carol's room. She was flailing her restrained arms wildly to rip out her breathing tubes.

Her face was literally beet red and she was drenched in sweat.

The nurse prompted me: "Should we push some Propofol to sedate her?"

I almost agreed with her reflexively. It wouldn't be long before she pulled the tube out. But a quick glance at the monitors showed that she was breathing quite well on her own. She didn't need the ventilator: "Wait, just pull the tube."

The respiratory therapist was uncertain: "Shouldn't we check with the attending?"

"No time! Let's do it."

Within minutes, the tube was out and Carol had a violent coughing fit. Her chest slowly stopped heaving as her breathing slowed down to a normal rate. She scowled at me accusingly. "*What* are you doing to me?"

There was a collective exhalation and the small congregation of nurses and respiratory therapists started to disperse.

I smiled. "Welcome back, Carol!"

Carol admitted that she sometimes dug into her old prescriptions when she had difficulty sleeping, but she didn't remember what happened after the Valium.

Two hours later, Ann sprinted past me and engulfed a bewildered Carol in a bear hug. Carol's blonde hair glinted in the sunlight streaming through the large window. Snowclad hills in the distance made for a dazzling backdrop. I ignored the irritable pager buzzing in my pocket to enjoy the moment.

Rounding took longer than usual that day. I had to explain my unilateral decision to extubate Carol and got a mild slap on the wrist for not asking an attending first. I didn't mind. It was worth it.

Before leaving for the day, I stopped by Carol's room. Patients are rarely discharged from the ICU, but Carol was far too well to be in a hospital now.

They were getting ready to leave. I bid them good luck with their Christmas party, which was now back on. Ann walked me out of the room.

"Hey," she said, "I never got to thank you."

The truth was that I was feeling pretty good about myself. My actions had directly made a difference in another human being's life. And yet, this obviously was not the first time. In big or small ways doctors tangibly affect the lives of patients under their care every day. The unrelenting pace of residency leaves us with little time to savor our little victories every day. Our failures, on the other hand, leave a lasting aftertaste. Carol's dramatic arc had refreshed my perspective. I felt new appreciation and gratitude to be part of such a consequential profession. I mattered!

"Oh, it's nothing," I protested with half-baked humility. "Just doing my job."

"This was the best Christmas gift ever," she said as she gave me a hug. It had been a hard four weeks, but in that moment, I knew that I had the best job in the world.

The Last Word

"Not pretty," I said with a wince.

Our team in the medical intensive care unit was looking at the CT scans of Raymond's abdomen. It looked like someone had used a bubble machine from a street fair to fill his belly with dozens of large bubbles. The radiologist's report was grim: the bubbles actually represented pockets of infection and they were growing in number.

Meg, my intern, offered to suck out fluid from one of those pockets to assess the progression of his infection. Even though this was the first month of her intern year, Meg was bold in thought and action. She had the answers to the questions I asked as well as the ones I didn't. Whereas many interns shrink from procedures, Meg sought them out eagerly.

So, I watched her as she cleaned Raymond's skin, injected local anesthetic, and smoothly inserted a needle into his abdomen. One look at the gray pus that filled her syringe confirmed our worst suspicions. The infection had taken a deep hold within Raymond's body. Without draining and breaking up the pockets, we would not be able to save him.

But Raymond didn't really care about the pockets in his belly, the blood in his stool, or the pus in our syringe. He had been lying in an ICU bed for almost a month now. He ached to sit in a chair. Unfortunately, a string of unfortunate events—critically low blood pressures and dangerous bleeds—had postponed the journey from bed to chair. Even now, his alertness waxed and waned. We were worried that he would tumble out of the chair and fracture a bone.

In the afternoons, I often heard his reedy voice through a crack in his door: "Chair…chair…chair…"

The surgeons swung by later in the day. They had seen the CT scan, and told us that surgery to remove the pockets was not an option.

We didn't disagree. Raymond's heart was delicate, his kidneys were functioning at a fraction of their capacity, and his liver was failing. He couldn't possibly survive the stress of a complicated abdominal surgery. We didn't have any options left.

With a heavy heart, Meg and I sat down with Tyrone, Raymond's son. Tyrone knew the details of his father's care well. We had been speaking on the phone every day.

"What did the surgeons say, doc?"

I looked at him, wishing I had a different answer.

"Tyrone, they can't fix the problem. He's not stable enough to handle the surgery."

"OK." He wrinkled his brow. "So, you're gonna keep sucking out the fluid and giving the antibiotics?"

"Honestly," I said gingerly, "I'm not sure that's going to help him. We can't kill the bacteria without removing the pockets."

Tyrone understood. I had warned him of this eventuality a few days ago.

"Is it time?"

"It is time."

Meg changed the code status in the chart. We stood outside Raymond's room and looked at him lying in his bed, his eyes closed. All of a sudden, his lips moved, and the ghost of a sound emerged: "Chair…chair…chair…"

Meg turned to me. "Does he have to lie down?"

I rubbed my chin. "He's high risk for a fall…"

"Does it really matter at this point? It's the one thing he asks clearly and consistently!"

I looked at her. I had never seen Meg so impassioned.

"Fine. Let's do it."

The nurses and the physical therapists weren't very happy about Meg's mission. I stood at the sidelines as she talked to four seasoned nurses. The conversation was heated at times, but she won them over in the end. Four of us gently guided Raymond out of bed and placed him in a recliner chair.

A strange paradox of residency life is that sometimes the work takes you away from the object of your exertions—the patient. Seeing Raymond recline comfortably in the chair, a white sheet covering his bulbous belly, I realized for the first time how tall he was. His eyes were kind and there was some salt and pepper in his sideburns. As our eyes met, I felt like I was meeting him for the first time.

As we stood by his chair, admiring our handiwork, Raymond looked up at us. He wanted to say something. I was half afraid that it would be "chair." Instead, he said, "Thank you."

The next day, without warning, blood started gushing out of Raymond's intestines. His blood pressure dropped. He was back in the bed with blood and medicines pouring into his veins. Despite our best efforts, the crimson tide refused to ebb. I called Tyrone.

Through sobs, he told me he was on the way and instructed me to allow a natural death. I promised him that there would be no pain.

Meg and I walked into Raymond's room together. One by one, we removed all unnecessary IV drips. He was back in bed now, piled high with blankets. The blood pressure cuff was blaring at us ominously.

I shut it off. The numbers did not matter now.

We sat by him and saw each breath become more labored than the one before. His eyes were closed. I wondered if he was conserving his energy for something. Was he waiting for someone? Was he waiting for something?

I asked, "Do you believe in heaven?"

"Yes," he murmured. The eyes remained closed.

I am not sure what prompted me to ask my next question: "Do you think you're going there?"

He nodded with his eyes still closed.

Meg joined in: "Would you like to pray?"

Another nod.

Meg stood up and leaned over him. She took his skeletal hands in hers. As if on cue, he opened his eyes and looked into hers.

Her voice quavering, Meg chanted, "Our father who art in heaven..."

He joined in. His voice had a deeper timbre than before. It was as if he knew that these would be his last lucid words.

I watched with wet cheeks as the doctor and the patient united in worship.

The tears I shed in that room were those of grief—a physician's sorrow at the imminent demise of a patient under his care. But they were also tears of pride as I watched my intern transcend her duties as a physician to fulfill those of a human. They were tears also of hope for this profession that we are so fortunate to call our own.

Urine Trouble

"So I faked a seizure…big deal!"

Harry threw his hands up, palm forward, as he confessed. He glowered at me, blue eyes wide with indignation behind chunky, framed glasses.

His Brooklyn accent was unmistakable, particularly when he asked for "wa-ta." With his disheveled gray hair, glasses, and rumpled tweed blazer, he reminded me of Woody Allen, if the great filmmaker had decided to boycott pants and smelled of urine.

"And I'd do it again too. They were just pissing me off, doc!"

"Who?" I asked. "The lawyers?"

"And the judge…the whole bunch of them."

"What did you do?"

"I just put my head back and said stuff like 'I'm dizzy…I can't see…help me!' Next thing I know I was in the hospital with a doctor whacking my knee with a hammer."

"Well, Harry, that's what happens when people think you're having a stroke or seizure."

"OK, so maybe I regret faking the seizure a little."

"And what happened to your pants?"

He glanced down at his bare thighs and looked nonplussed, as if he had noticed for the first time the pants-free landscape of his lower extremities.

"To tell you the truth, I really couldn't say."

Bit by bit, I pieced the story together. Three weeks ago, Harry woke up and started his regular pilgrimage to the local Dunkin Donuts. He wasn't completely sure if he was wearing pants at this point in the day. Halfway to the coffee shop, he realized that he had forgotten to use the toilet at home. Considering an alley wall a reasonable substitute, he proceeded to relieve his bladder. Much to his dismay, an unmarked police car had been using the very same alley as a good stakeout spot for graffiti artists and other unsavory characters.

And so he wound up in court, where a social worker and judge began to talk about his capacity to care for himself.
Harry had a pattern of behavioral problems that raised concerns about cognitive impairment. He had no family of his own and no social support apart from a few friends. The judge wanted to assign a lawyer to make Harry's medical and financial decisions for him. Harry didn't like this talk one bit and faked his seizure to get out of a tricky situation.

The judge ordered for him to be held in the hospital for care until long-term plans could be made for him. After the neurologists realized that he was in no imminent danger, he was sent to the medicine ward as a "social admit." Now, regardless of his wishes or mine, he was stuck in the hospital under my care.

I had cared for patients in Harry's social situation before. Often, patients like him end up in the hospital for weeks, even months, as they wait for the slow cogs of bureaucracy to turn. Patients like Harry don't understand why they need help, and often hurl abuse at the physicians and nurses who watch over them.

Residents don't love the situation much more than the patients. There's no diagnosis to be made, no test to be ordered, and no prescription to be given.

Watching over patients like Harry resembles the work of prison wardens more than it does that of physicians.

"Another rock," I said to my attending physician. I was using the slang doctors use for patients like Harry, since moving them out of the hospital often proves a Sisyphean task. I am not fond of the term, but it has become something of a shorthand.

The attending smiled wryly. "We're running the geology service, huh?"

As far as rocks go, Harry was never boring. I kept my visits brief because he didn't need anything by way of medical attention. Still, I loved peeking into his room as I passed by, because there was always something unusual going on inside.

I kept a mental diary of Harry's escapades.

Day 2: Lying on his back with his blazer rolled up under his head as a pillow. Legs were crossed with insouciance and his feet were tapping out an unheard rhythm. Studying the ceiling. Still no pants.

Day 3: Giving my intern detailed instructions on tuning a violin. Still no pants.

Day 4: Arguing with his nurse about his right to forego pants. Invoking the first amendment.

Day 5: Scribbling furiously in a notebook. Explained himself when he caught me staring: "Practicing long division." Now wearing blue scrub pants.

By the end of the week, I was conscious of a steadily intensifying smell of urine in Harry's room. I wrinkled my nose during one of my routine peek-ins and started to step out, only to be accosted by Patty, Harry's nurse.

Patty had a lovely Jamaican accent and a rich laugh, but she withheld all her charm from doctors who wasted her time. Right then, she wasn't too pleased with me.

"Doc, he smells too much."

"Has he taken a shower?"

"Not since he got here. He keeps talking about violating the Geneva Convention."

I sniggered.

Patty was not amused. "What are you going to do about it, doc? It's too much!"

Inspiration struck: "OK, how about this? If he showers, I'll personally take him to the healing garden after we sign out to the night team."

Harry readily agreed to this deal and hurriedly took a shower.

The healing garden was located on the seventh floor of our hospital and offered lovely views of the city and its surroundings.

Wind chimes tinkled, a brook babbled, and leaves rustled. Many patients and hospital personnel found a modicum of serenity in the garden.

Harry loved it.

He gazed out in wonderment at the city in the foreground with its buildings, traffic lights, and cars, and marveled at the ragged hills in the distance. He even caught a glimpse of the Long Island Sound.

After spending a few minutes pointing out landmarks, he quieted down as the sun sank behind the hills, bleeding a vermillion hue into the sky. I stood next to him and shared the view. Every fiber in his body yearned to escape from this hospital-prison. Every fiber in my body wanted to free him. Neither of us spoke a word.

After a few minutes, he turned away from the sunset and began pottering around the garden. I sat down and gazed at the darkening sky.

As the moon grew more prominent, I found myself asking the same questions I ask myself every time I take care of a patient like Harry.

"Don't we all make bad decisions now and then? What does one have to do to lose control over one's life? Am I right to keep Harry shackled in a hospital?"

My musings were interrupted by a couple of loud gasps behind me. I whipped around to find two women shrinking in horror from Harry, their hands clasped to their mouths in apoplectic mortification. One was trying in vain to cover her young daughter's eyes.

Oblivious to them, Harry was standing atop a faux-boulder. A tuft of his hair was billowing in the breeze and his blue scrub pants were around his ankles. He was waving excitedly at me with one hand and using the other to direct a parabolic arc of amber urine into the babbling brook.

Nails and Screw-ups

I twirled the nail clippers invitingly. "The usual?"

He smiled bashfully.

Michael was one of my favorite patients at the VA (Veterans Affairs) clinic. We had dealt with everything from his depression to his high blood pressure in the one year that I had known him.

Being morbidly obese, he wasn't able to reach his toes. When he struggled to find a podiatrist to trim his unruly nails on a regular basis, I started clipping them for him.

His sallow toenails had become rough and gnarled like a weathered oak. To cut them, I had to grab the nail clipper with both hands, scrunch my eyes shut, and squeeze with all my might until my knuckles whitened and my forearms quivered. With resounding clicks, like musket shots, his nails would ricochet off into unexplored crannies of the clinic room.

The nail clipping took time and gave us plenty of time to chat. He told me of his time as a medic in the military. I told him about how weird it was to have people call me "Doc." He told me of his wild life in the summer of love— not something I had expected, based on his venerable appearance now. I told him that he needed to take a trip away from his musty apartment. He agreed and spoke wistfully of Arizona, where his favorite cousin lived. I urged him to save up for a ticket. He did so.

Consequently, I was dismayed when Jack, my clinic preceptor called me as I was waiting to board an Air India flight at JFK: "Pranay, this is Jack. Michael was just admitted to the university center with chest pain."

"Damn it," I cursed under my breath as my laptop sputtered to life, "I screwed up."

At a visit two weeks ago, he had seemed less energetic than usual. When I asked him about his haggard appearance, he mentioned that he had been feeling light-headed and had come close to passing out. A quick review of his medicine list provided the answer: he was on too many blood-pressure (BP) medications because of his history of multiple heart attacks. Indeed, his BP was too low when I checked it in the office.

I stopped one of his BP meds immediately. When I called him the next day, he felt a bit better. On a return visit the day before my flight, he reported still having some episodes of light-headedness, so I lowered the dose of his Metoprolol, another medication for BP. Little did I know how tenuous his circulation was. Within a day, he experienced a chest pain akin to his previous heart attacks and was rushed to the university medical center.

Michael had been cared for at the VA for years and had never been to the university hospital. I logged into the university medical record system and quickly typed up a summary of the medication adjustment.

After signing the note, I reread my last sentence: "In summary, the chest pain is likely associated with a down-titration of his blood pressure medications that were also playing an anti-anginal role."

That verbose sentence, filled with sterile language, stated one simple fact: "Damn it, I screwed up."

I returned from India in two weeks and immediately called Michael. His voice sounded uncharacteristically flat on the phone. When I pointed this out, he told me that he was depressed about his hospital bills.

Even though Michael was a veteran and a Medicare beneficiary, a perfect storm of administrative issues and a billing snafu had left him holding a sizable bill. He was now dipping into his savings.

"I guess Arizona won't be happening now…"

I was outraged. "They can't do this." I stormed into Jack's office, my clinic supervisor, and told him that I wouldn't tolerate this bureaucratic bullshit. The guy had served his country and deserved better. Jack and I pleaded Michael's case to social workers, care coordinators, and several officials. No dice.

Michael would quite literally be paying for my mistake. Overwhelmed, I sat down heavily on a chair in Jack's office and put my head in my hands. I had just started gaining some confidence in my clinical skills. Now I was confronted with the stark ugliness of my incompetence.

Jack watched me for a few seconds as I massaged my temples and rocked back and forth.

"Are you OK?"

"It's just…I screwed up. This is all *my* fault."

Jack considered me over his rimless glasses. Despite his gray hair, he looks ageless, and it would be hard for the casual observer to know that he had been a doctor much longer than I have been alive. He matched the energy and enthusiasm of youth with the patience and perspective of later years.

"Think about it this way: you have learned something about him now, haven't you?"

Instead of lecturing or punishing me, Jack encouraged me to continue my crusade of solving Michael's financial troubles. He and I started calling the local congresswoman and some veterans' organizations for help. Finally, we connected Michael to two local veteran organizations that neutralized his medical debts.

And yet, I reckoned the damage was done. Even though Jack had been so understanding, I figured Michael would not see things so charitably.

No longer would he entrust his body to a young upstart like me. The guilt and shame became an albatross around my neck. So, I was grateful when I was not available for his next visit to the VA. He met with Jack instead.

I could run, but I couldn't hide. Within two months, Michael was sitting across me in the clinic room. I looked at him awkwardly.

"Hey."

"Hi."

I looked at the man, not knowing what to say. "How've you been?" I ventured.

"Oh…you know…" he responded in his demure way.

My heart was beating quickly and my ears felt warm. I couldn't bring myself to meet his eyes, so I stared at my computer screen instead.

For some reason, I kept thinking about the advice lawyers often given to young doctors: "Never admit fault, even if you've made a mistake." This dictum has never sat quite right with me. If we take credit for the hundreds of things that we do well every day, how can we not also take the responsibility for the times we bungle and fumble? How can our patients trust us if we avert our eyes in the aftermath of missteps?

I turned my chair toward him and looked at him directly. He peered back through his thick glasses. His eyes were kind and his hands were comfortably interlaced on top of his protuberant belly. I was conscious of a deep affection for the man, a protectiveness I had not felt before. I wanted him to be happy and healthy. Somehow, an apology seemed the only possible first step. I couldn't keep it within me anymore.

"Michael, I am sorry!"

"Whatever for?"

"I never should have fiddled with your meds! I feel responsible for your hospitalizations and those bills. It was cavalier of me."

He seemed taken aback by my outburst and was silent for a few seconds.

"That's OK. I know you were trying to help."

Relief washed over me. I sank back into the chair and realized how tense my muscles had been. He noticed and smiled. I grinned back as I felt a weight being lifted from my shoulders. With a simple sentence and a smile, he had de-albatrossed me.

"So, what can I do for you today?"

He pointed to his toes. "The usual."

A Burden I Was Happy to Bear

"He was thrashing around all night," the nurse reported, "but the oxycodone knocked him out around three a.m."

Sedated by his pain medications, Ted slept despite the rhythmic ruckus of his breathing machine and his assortment of blaring monitors. He would later complain that he never felt quite rested in the hospital.

While awake, his gaze often lingered on a snapshot that captured him in the past: full of laughter and radiant joy with his little granddaughter, Tara. The grandfather in the photo—muscular, mischievous—barely resembled the emaciated elder in the bed who silently mouthed short answers to my questions. The twinkle in his eyes was gone.

He had come to the hospital for cancer chemotherapy, but he deteriorated, and within a few weeks he needed support from a breathing machine to survive. The breathing tube and his weakened immune system begat further pneumonias and the ventilator became a fixture in his life. Soon, he developed irreversible kidney failure and began needing dialysis as well.

By the time I met him, he had been on a ventilator in the ICU for eleven months. Multiple attempts to get him off the breathing machine had been foiled by infections and assorted organ dysfunctions.

Most patients stop needing breathing machines within days, but there are some patients who remain ventilator dependent for weeks, months, or even years, thus acquiring the diagnosis of "chronic critical illness."

For patients like Ted, who have worsening multi-organ failure, mechanical ventilation serves to keep them alive, but is powerless to return them to their former healthy selves. Additional therapies such as tube feeds, dialysis, and antibiotics also prolong the dying process from hours to months or even years.

Ted, like many patients with chronic critical illness, had to endure them all: breathing tubes, feeding tubes, injections, pain, thirst, nausea, and recurrent infections.

He did this in hopes of a miracle that could end his dependence on machines and custodial caretakers, in hopes that he could go home, in hopes that he could play with Tara once again. His hopes rose and fell with the daily fluctuations in his clinical status. To me, he was the embodiment of Nietzsche's words: "He who has a Why to live for can bear almost any How."

His prolonged illness was taking its toll on his family members. His wife, Mary, spent her days shuttling between work at her car dealership and Ted's room. "When he gets worse and I am not here by his side," she once told me, "I can't shake the feeling that it's my fault...that I could have stopped it if I had been around." She was a petite woman with a mane of ginger hair and a penchant for enormous earrings. She left Ted with visible reluctance every night around 11:00 p.m. "A part of my soul never leaves this room," she explained.

Caring for patients with chronic critical illness is draining for physicians and nurses too. In our short stints in the ICU, physicians cannot always build the strong relationships with patients and families that can help us jointly come to terms with such grim prognoses.

Instead, like many residents before me, I catch myself going through the motions of care perfunctorily—doing physical exams, rounding, and writing prescriptions despite knowing that I cannot give back to my patients their identities and their lives before their tragic illnesses.

In such situations, I feel trapped and guilty: this is not the doctoring I was prepared to do. Physicians and nurses study and train hard for the joy of alleviating pain and mitigating the tyranny of disease—not to prolong the inexorable decay of irreparable bodies.

I had only been taking care of Ted for three days when the oncology fellow approached me with bad news.

"Light chains are elevated. Chemotherapy has failed." Ted's cancer was back despite multiple rounds of chemotherapy. We shared the news with Ted and Mary.

Mary remained resolute: "So what will we try next?"

"There's no effective therapy left to try," admitted the oncology fellow. He paused to let the words sink in and looked down at his hands sheepishly. Sitting next to him, I knew we were unified in that moment by a familiar frustration: *After eight years of schooling and degrees worth a quarter of a million dollars, why do I not have more to offer?*

Once the shock had abated a little, we discussed the possibility of transitioning to comfort care, explaining that, in the absence of treatments for his cancer, we were prolonging his life with mechanical ventilation, dialysis, and antibiotics for his recurrent and increasingly drug-resistant pneumonias.

Didn't he just want to be comfortable? To drift into a deep sleep and be free of the pain and the frustration?

I strained to read Ted's lips as he mouthed his response. Sunrays streamed through the window and the bright light glanced off his face. His face seemed puffy, but his eyes were not droopy today; they were fixed firmly on me. I only understood him on the third repetition: "I am scared of dying. I don't want to kill myself."

I placed my hand on his right leg, noting for the first time just how shriveled his once-mighty calves had become. It was time to say the words that no physician liked to utter: "Ted, we cannot stop you from dying. But," I added with as much conviction I could muster, "we can help you die on your own terms."

He remained unmoved and was getting tired with the effort of conversation. I began wondering if he even had the capacity to make this difficult decision. Mary requested to speak to me separately. Though she agreed with me, she couldn't bear to withdraw life support. "I know he's dying, but I don't want to kill him. I'll never forgive myself and neither will our children."

I knew I was asking too much of them. The decision to stop therapy is inordinately difficult. For many people, terminating care is tantamount to giving up on their dying kin or, worse, murdering them. Those who make this courageous decision often struggle with doubt and guilt for many years. After all, these patients have pulses, warm skin, and tears. Patients who have to decide for themselves often equate stopping life support with suicide. They worry about letting their families down. Some even consider it an unforgivable sin. Who is to say that they are right or wrong?

Inappropriate cultural defaults within our health-care system force people into chronic critical illness. Life-sustaining therapies are frequently started quickly without clearly set expectations, goals, or defined endpoints. Escalation of care occurs algorithmically. When even the most aggressive therapies fail to change the course of the disease, patients and their families are often asked to make the difficult decision about stopping or continuing care. Putting them in this position seems cruel.

Cessation of care usually occurs in two ways: either the patient or family decides to forego life-sustaining therapy, or the patient becomes so sick that medical and surgical therapies stop working.

Physicians are often torn between the principles of autonomy and beneficence in cases like Ted's. As physicians, we know that the patients are suffering. We know that their chances of returning to the life they desire are non-existent. We know that this is a difficult decision. Should we respect their right to self-determination and help them continue this difficult existence until they decide to stop?

Or should we volunteer ourselves as stewards, relieve them of the burden of the decision, and guide them to a comfortable and dignified death?

Potent arguments can be made for both sides.

But perhaps the choice doesn't have to be binary. My attending physician found a middle path. He sat down next to Ted.

"I know the weight of this decision is unbearable. Would you allow me to take that burden away from you? It is my job, and I know I can live with the consequences of the decision."

Ted and Mary said they would think about it.

To share this decisional burden requires confidence, integrity, and a deep respect for the patient. Our patients will never share their burden unless they trust us. Trust takes time and demands good communication.

I had discovered an important role and suddenly felt empowered. Over the next two weeks, I got to know the man beyond the chart.

Ted and Mary loved tennis. She was better than him in their prime. He had been a detective and told me about the murder case he had solved in sixteen hours. Ted's brother was doing well in his Alcoholic Anonymous (AA) program. His daughter had been putting off her wedding until he could attend it. Tara's kindergarten escapades made me convulse with laughter. Laughter, an almost foreign entity in the room, seemed to have obtained a temporary visa. For me, these trust-building interactions became as important as placing venous catheters or reviewing labs.

Thanks to a strong team effort from a battalion of nurses, respiratory therapists, physical therapists, occupational therapists, aides, and doctors, Ted began tolerating minimal ventilator settings and had stood on his feet for the first time in weeks.

But the progress evanesced overnight when worsening breathlessness and thick purulent secretions announced yet another pneumonia. Mary was visibly crestfallen. I had a light workload that day so I suggested taking a walk to the healing garden in our hospital. It was a windy day and rain seemed imminent. The wind chime produced a surprisingly calming tune even though it was flailing around as though attacked by a dozen invisible six-year-olds.

I asked: "Should we go back in?"

"Let's sit for a few minutes."

Below us, we saw a white bird with gray wingtips—a seagull, perhaps—prominent in the dark sky. He was beating his wings furiously to counter the howling wind that engulfed him. Powerful though his strokes must have been, they were powerless against the formidable force of the wind that surrounded us. His wings seemed to move in slow motion as he hung stationary in the air.

There was something tragicomic about his inability to move. I sensed that Mary too was rooting for the bird, the clear underdog. After thirty seconds, his flapping slowed down and, quite abruptly, he swooped down onto the monolithic gray garage below him. There, he appeared to brace himself behind a four-foot wall.

"He looks tired," said Mary.

"Yes." I agreed.

The inevitable words came out now: "What should we do?"

Ted and Mary at long last shared their difficult burden with us. It was a weight we felt privileged to bear as we watched him drift into an undisturbed final deep sleep.

Yogesh

The chief resident's face quivered as he told us about Yogesh's terminal brain cancer.

In polite society, words like cancer and tumor are spoken in hushed voices. Residents utter them matter-of-factly during sign-out, with practiced sensitivity in family meetings, or even triumphantly in didactic sessions.

This was different. We sat silently, lacking the courage to look anyone else in the eye. The stillness was punctuated by irrepressible sobs.

Yogesh, "Yogi bear" to his friends, wore the white coat better than most. His impeccably worded notes remain in the charts of scores of patients as testament to his professional excellence.

As a medical student and then resident, he had cared for patients from New Haven to Nepal, from Seattle to South Africa, from Guilford to Ghana. As chief resident, he held us to the highest standards. No one was surprised when he matched into a staggeringly prestigious fellowship program. It simply did not compute that this sagacious young physician was abruptly forced to confront his mortality.

Residency program directors all over the country profess that their programs are families. Working together through adversity to save lives rapidly builds lasting bonds. Yogesh's illness put that claim to the test and we passed muster. We raised money. We curated Spotify lists. We cooked vegetarian food. Yogesh's hospital room became a menagerie of plush animals. One of us even hoisted a whimsical tribute to Yogi on a highway billboard. Never have I been so proud of my residency community.

Yogesh's illness was a testament to the fragility of our identities and our elaborate life plans.

Asked what he or she wants to do, no resident would ever answer "residency." Our plans involve research, teaching, families, and more. Our plans span decades beyond the present. Medical school, residency, and fellowships are just dues that must be paid. The prospect of those plans—our future—dissolving like a powerless lump of sugar, is horrific.

In his final weeks, Yogesh took to writing occasional updates. I have read and reread his words to understand how he dealt with the sudden dissolution of his dreams. The words he left are full of the wisdom and beauty with which he authored the final chapter of his life.

A physician to the end, he learned a new lesson in empathy upon being diagnosed with brain cancer himself: "…did my patients ever know just how I truly never knew what they were going through?" We learned a new lesson too. Many of us had never experienced a cancer diagnosis this way. I know that the tears I choked back and the tears that I couldn't shall continue to irrigate my empathy for suffering patients, families, and friends.

In a subsequent update, he articulated the loneliness of disease: "With everyone around me in the ensuing days, despite fake-neck tattoos in solidarity of my planned biopsy, I was alone. In the uniqueness of the experience, no one knew my reality. But what was more unique, was being gracefully on the receiving end of life's work and passion. A tree branch being visited by birds with no agenda other than to share what comes natural."

Many of us cloak our vulnerabilities in the guise of strength or so-called "professionalism." The poetry of Yogesh's words is rare. His willingness to share his vulnerabilities is rarer still. Eventually, the grim reaper will catch up with us all. I pray that I can show as much gumption and grace when that moment comes.

I often sent Yogesh little jokes, tokens of my affection to brighten his day. He usually responded with very few words or a singular emoji. Weakened by chemotherapy and radiation, I expected that he couldn't possibly do much more.

Always full of surprises, he sent this touching missive: "In my silent, post-radiation and chemo afternoons, I can literally feel everyone's affection. I now know that what we think, our concern for others, eventually makes it to its intended target. I know. And so I wonder, how I got so lucky, to lay in my silent afternoons basking in all your affection."

In a quirky Etsy store, I found a pin with Yogi bear scampering with a picnic hamper. That pin now adorns the lapel of my white coat. It serves as a touchstone that reminds me daily of Yogesh's empathy, vulnerability, and grace. On bad days, when the future looks bleak, it reminds me that Yogesh touched hundreds of lives in his all-too-short life.

While my plans span decades, it takes only a few minutes to care for a suffering soul and make a difference. Even as residents we have those opportunities every day. Even as residents we are fortunate to lead lives of immense consequence.

The Yogi bear pin also reassures me that I am part of a beautiful community that will catch me if I stumble. To steal from Yogesh: "who will possibly deny, that despite everything, everything is perfect. I am honestly the luckiest. To be right here, right now."

An Intern Writes to His Future Self

Dear future Pranay,

I'm not sure where life has taken you—you might be a serious senior resident physician, a frazzled fellow, or—maybe—living your dream of being an eccentric train conductor with an affinity for shoe polish and writing novels.

I am writing this letter to you on the last day of intern year. Wherever life has brought you, take five minutes, sit back, put your feet up, stop being distracted by the passing scenery on the Northeast regional, and think about your humble beginnings.

How far you have come from the fresh-faced, bow-tie-wearing, revoltingly cheerful fellow who stumbled anytime he had to introduce himself!

The first few days in the hospital were so gruesome that they'd have been conducted off-stage in any respectable Greek tragedy. People actually expected you to know stuff. What a notion!

Sure, you had gained vague ideas of what PTs and PTTs were in med school, but what were you to do when gimlet-eyed nurses asked you to adjust heparin drips? Need I remind you of your frequent urge to dive into a corner and impersonate a HIPAA compliant dustbin until people left you alone?

And why, in the name of all that is digital, did we have to pre-round and present every patient every morning? Was there a celestial curse upon our attendings and residents that blinded them to readily available information on the very computers they pushed around?

The only thing worse than supervisors ignoring the information before them was supervisors entranced by it. When around supervisors thus transfixed, presentations felt like ancient rituals necessary to stave off famine.

Pimping, a weaponized version of the Socratic method, was mercifully minimal, but sometimes it did feel like a form of advanced interrogation that Dick Cheney would support. What on earth is Throck-Morton sign anyway? It didn't help that the IQ-depleting gaze of some attendings reduced your intellect to that of a salamander who had had a difficult birth.

And then came the notes—the scourge of every intern. You probably spent more time doctoring your notes than your patients. Does every patient really need Shakespearean prose written about them daily?

To be or not to be...full code.

The drug seeker doth protest too much, methinks!

The course of true love and MICU admissions never did run smooth.

Brevity is the soul of wit…and the key to going home early.

The better part of valor is Vanc/Zosyn.

The cacophony of pagers, so integral to the intern experience, wreaked havoc on your psyche. Your best friends developed the dreaded pager-traumatic stress disorder, with dreadful flares during backup rotations. Symptoms included jumping at small sounds, checking the pager obsessively for missed pages, and compulsively bringing your pager into the shower.

Each page filled you with a nameless dread, especially at first, and you asked deep existential questions about why you got yourself into this mess in the first place? You had fleeting regrets about passing up on a graduate degree in gender studies or English literature.

Most dangerous, of course, was the ever-present threat of crippling cynicism. Inappropriate ICU care, overly optimistic code statuses, needless admissions, helplessness before cancer, and unprecedented exhaustion eroded your spirit. You became the gruff curmudgeon given to slurred soliloquies about life, the universe, and the medical-industrial complex.

There is probably no escaping the malaise associated with internship. Doctors, like Rome, are not built in a day. But slowly and imperceptibly, over the course of the year, you and your friends became competent physicians.

Before you knew it, notes were done before rounds, pages lost their terror, and you learned to make even the most solemn attendings and nurses snort with laughter. Managing chest pain, shortness of breath, and electrolyte problems became surprisingly ordinary. With increasing competence, your initial wretchedness and inadequacy gave way to renewed joy in medicine. Most importantly, your humanism, ethics, and general sense of optimism survived intern year.

You couldn't have done it without compassionate co-interns who listened to the aforementioned soliloquies and salved your wounds with kind words or the occasional frozen yogurt. Almost every day, you were rescued by residents and attendings in shining armor— well, bleached white coats at any rate.

They taught you to manage sick patients, listened to your rants, took annoying tasks off your hands and respected you. They spared you from "paying" most of your supposed "dues" because they remembered their own struggles with heparin drips, "hypernotemia," and pager-traumatic stress disorder.

I write to you now, at the end of my intern year, to refresh your memory and dispel recall bias. If you are currently supervising interns, remember your humble origins and cut them slack. Do the things that made you adore your favorite residents and attendings.

Take a genuine interest in your interns as human beings and trainees. Fake curiosity is cloying.

When you teach, do so to improve their knowledge, not to showcase yours. Respect their intellect and don't be embarrassed to learn from them. Remember that interns prefer to work with human beings, not demigods.

Pay attention on rounds and make eye contact. The occasional encouraging smile or wink goes a long way. Make them feel like valuable members of the team, not chroniclers of your escapades. If you see them struggling with something you also struggled with, share your experience candidly to remind them that they aren't alone, and that there is hope.

Oh…also, donuts and coffee don't hurt on the weekends.

If, however, you ended up becoming a train conductor, enjoy the scenery, polish your shoes, and write a good novel.

Yours truly,

Pranay

A Final Word

If you've gotten this far, I must thank you profusely. I hope the book made you snort with laughter and sob with heartache—to go without those two extremes of emotions is to not live at all. I also hope that it was quick. Nobody likes a long-winded gasbag. Most of all, I hope you choose to find joy.

It would be remiss of me to end this book without pointing out that mental health services for health professionals are crucial. In the throes of depression, a common occupational hazard in medicine, a positive outlook is often insufficient. Don't be afraid to ask for help.

When I published an introduction to this book online, some disgruntled readers accused me of "settling" for scraps of joys. They crackled with the fury of a thousand suns and were allegedly prepared to burn the system down and rebuild it. More power to them.

Although I am not likely to pick up a torch or a pitchfork anytime soon, I concur that systemic changes are imperative to decrease the structural violence done against our mental and physical wellness. Indeed, leaders like Dr. Christine Sinsky exhort physicians to audaciously pursue joy in practice through implementable changes in the way we structure our practice of medicine.

I would also like to remind individuals of the burn-and-rebuild persuasion that no system is perfect. And the skill of finding and savoring everyday tidbits of joy will likely still be useful even beyond their professional lives.

Now put this book away and go be joyful!

Attributions

"The Best Christmas Gift I Ever Gave" and "A Burden I was Happy to Bear" were first published in *The Huffington Post*. "An Intern Writes to His Future Self" was first published on the *Kevin MD* blog. "Yogesh" and "The Last Word" were first published in *The Beeson Beat*.

Acknowledgments

My wife and I have a ritual that precedes all (well, most!) of our meals together. We say our thanks for the good things, big and small, going on in our lives that day. It's a good ritual that has made us grateful for our lot in life. Some people come up often.

I often thank Lisa Sanders, Marcia Childress, Mark Siegel, Anna Reisman, Rebecca Slotkin, Merilyn Varghese, Jack Hughes and Bryan Brown for their consistently thoughtful edits without which this book would lack substance and style.

I often thank the Khanal family for allowing me to share Yogesh's important story.

I often thank Barry Zaret and Abraham Verghese who give nascent physician-writers like me an ideal to approximate.

I often thank Jill Grimes for giving me the courage to pursue independent publishing.

I often thank Seth Michelson, who taught me to write in the first place.

I always thank Anandmayee Sinha, Prem Kumar Sinha, Pranav Sinha, and Bhagya Saxena, who filled my youth (and now adult life) with joy.

And I am eternally grateful to my long-suffering wife, Anne Liu, who is my everything.

Cover Design

My darling cousin Mimansa helped me design the cover of this book.

The photograph on the front cover features sunlight on a cloudy day streaming through the strands in a small piece of medical gauze. It seemed befitting for a book searching for joy and meaning in medicine.

About the Author

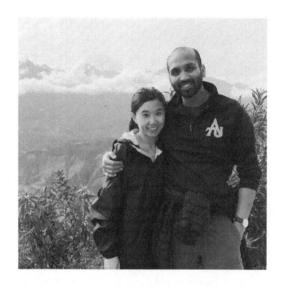

Pranay grew up in India under the watchful eye of doctor parents while suffering the tyranny of his older brother. He came to America for college and graduated *summa cum laude* from Adelphi University with a BS in Biology. He attended medical school at the University of Virginia where he was inducted into the Gold Humanism Honor Society and received the prestigious Edgar F. Shannon award. Thereafter, he completed his residency in Internal Medicine at Yale-New Haven Hospital where he became involved in efforts to improve resident wellness. His essays on physician wellness and humanism appeared in the *New York Times*, *Huffington Post*, and the *Los Angeles Times*. Pranay is now training in the Boston University Infectious Diseases Fellowship program. He lives with his wife (formerly his supervising resident) and his dog (Shih-Tzu-Samiasis) in Boston, MA.

Early Praise for *In the Space Between Moments*

"A trainee doctor combats burnout with heartening stories of how medical professionals make a difference in patients' lives.

Debut author Sinha wrote these seven concise, well-crafted pieces while he was in internal medicine residency training at Yale New Haven Hospital...The author is always cognizant of how comedy and tragedy alternate, or even overlap, in emergency situations.... These punchy essays (five of which have been previously published on websites) glisten with just-right details, dialogue, and characterization.... The only problem with the book? It's too short—let's hope a few more years in practice will give the author sufficient material for a full-length work. Prescription: Read. Laugh. Cry. Repeat."

Kirkus Reviews

"Pranay Sinha has written a poignant, yet uplifting book that illuminates the sacred and trusting relationship between the patient and doctor. He is a masterful storyteller... the words spring up from the pages and the imagery evoked left my intellect a bit jolted on occasion but my heart feeling bigger every time. It is a must read for all of us privileged to serve in this truly magnificent and healing profession "

> Sanjiv Chopra MD MACP,
>
> Professor of Medicine
>
> Harvard Medical School

"These lovely and moving essays capture and explore difficult and emotional moments between doctors and patients. Dr. Sinha presents these narratives -- including one about a fellow resident's death -- with humility, respect, wit, and plenty of heart."

> Anna Reisman, MD
>
> Associate Professor of Medicine
>
> Yale School of Medicine

"Dr. Sinha beautifully unveils the powerful relationships that fuel the heart of medicine in this intentionally succinct collection of essays. I read it cover to cover in one sitting...and so will you, because you won't want to set it down! Senior pre-med students should be inspired (and motivated to plow through biochemistry and med school applications). Med students and young doctors in training will feel supported and encouraged to look beyond the lab numbers and differential diagnoses in their own patients, recharged by these touching stories."

Jill Grimes, MD FAAFP

Family Medicine Physician

Clinical Instructor

UMass Medical School

Made in the USA
Middletown, DE
25 July 2020

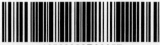